How To Lower Your Blood Pressure Naturally

A Guide To Lower Your Blood Pressure Without Prescription Drugs ,Medication Using Natural Remedies

By

Ella Anderson

TABLE OF CONTENT

Chapter 8: Monitoring And Maintaining Blood Pressure

Introduction

Keeping our bodies in tune with the rhythm of life is a symphony of choices, actions and perceptions. This comprehensive guide is your compass on your transformational journey to achieve and maintain optimal blood pressure levels through a natural, holistic approach.

High blood pressure or high blood pressure affects millions of people worldwide and is a major risk factor for cardiovascular disease.

In our busy modern lives, it's important to find a balance that promotes a healthy cardiovascular system. This e-book is more than just a collection of strategies.

This is an invitation to adopt a lifestyle that is in harmony with your body's natural rhythms.

This ebook covers the art and science of lowering blood pressure naturally.

From understanding everything about blood pressure to lifestyle adjustments, nutrition, stress management and more.

As you explore the web, this guide becomes your road map to sustainable health.

Our approach is not a quick fix or a temporary fix.

Rather, it is based on the belief that the choices we make every day have a significant impact on our health.

" How To Lower Your Blood Pressure Naturally" allows you to make conscious decisions and develop habits that align with your body's innate wisdom.

As you begin this journey, remember that each small step adds up to the symphony of a healthy and balanced life.

Let this guide be your companion, providing information, practical advice and a holistic perspective on managing blood pressure naturally.

Are you ready to adapt your lifestyle, nourish your body and unlock the transformative power of your overall health?

Start your journey.

Chapter 1
Understanding Blood Pressure

Understanding blood pressure is essential when researching natural ways to lower blood pressure. Blood pressure is the force with which blood pushes against the walls of blood vessels as the heart pumps blood throughout the body.

It is measured in millimeters of mercury (mmHg) and is made up of two values: systolic blood pressure (the force when the heart contracts) and diastolic blood pressure (the force when the heart rests between beats).

Healthy blood pressure values are usually around 120/80 mmHg. However, consistently high levels can lead to health problems, including cardiovascular problems.

Now let's learn how to lower blood pressure naturally.

Diet options:
Reduce sodium intake: High sodium levels can cause water retention and high blood pressure.
Maintain a diet low in processed foods and high in fresh fruits and vegetables.

Potassium-rich foods: Potassium helps balance sodium levels, so increase your intake of potassium-rich foods like bananas, oranges, spinach, and sweet potatoes.

Physical activity:

Aerobic exercise: Regular aerobic exercise, such as brisk walking, jogging or cycling, can have a significant effect on blood pressure.
Try to get at least 150 minutes of moderate-intensity exercise per week.
Weight Management:

Maintaining a healthy weight: Being overweight puts stress on the cardiovascular system and causes high blood pressure.
A balanced diet and regular exercise can help you manage your weight.
Reduces stress:

Mindfulness and relaxation techniques: Chronic stress can cause high blood pressure.

Manage your stress levels effectively by incorporating activities such as mindfulness exercises, deep breathing exercises and yoga.

Limit alcohol consumption and quit smoking:

Moderate alcohol consumption: Excessive alcohol consumption can increase blood pressure.

Please also consider moderation or abstinence.

Quit smoking: Smoking damages blood vessels and raises blood pressure.

Quitting smoking has a positive effect on your overall health as well as your blood pressure.

Enough sleep:

Prioritize quality sleep: Lack of sleep or poor quality sleep can cause high blood pressure.

To support overall cardiovascular health, aim for 7 to 9 hours of quality sleep each night.

Herbal Supplements:

Explore natural remedies: Certain herbs, such as hibiscus, garlic, and olive leaf, have been shown to lower blood pressure.

However, you should consult your doctor before taking these supplements.

It is important to understand that the natural approach combines these lifestyle changes.
It's not about making drastic changes overnight, it's about adopting lasting habits that contribute to a healthy lifestyle.
Regular monitoring, along with these natural interventions, can help people control their blood pressure overall.
user

Chapter 2
Lifestyle Changes

Lifestyle adjustments play an important role in lowering blood pressure naturally. These changes are not only effective, but promote long-term, sustainable cardiovascular health.

Let's take a look at some lifestyle changes that can help lower your blood pressure naturally.

Dietary changes:

Focus on a balanced diet.
Eat a diet rich in fruits, vegetables, whole grains, and lean protein.

Provides essential nutrients and helps maintain a healthy weight.

The DASH Diet: The Dietary Approaches to Stop High Blood Pressure (DASH) is a well-researched eating plan that has been shown to lower blood pressure.

Limit processed foods: Processed and packaged foods are high in sodium. Advising people to choose fresh, whole foods and prepare them at home can significantly reduce their sodium intake.
Read labels: Teach people to read food labels and learn about the hidden sodium in different foods.

Regular physical activity:

Aerobic exercise: Regular aerobic exercise, such as walking, running, swimming or cycling, improves cardiovascular health.
Try to get at least 150 minutes of moderate-intensity exercise per week.

Strength Training: Including strength training can help you improve your overall health and maintain a healthy weight.
Weight Management:

Body Mass Index (BMI): Discuss the importance of achieving and maintaining a healthy BMI.

Even a small weight loss can have a significant impact on blood pressure.

Portion control: Educate people about portion sizes and mindful eating to prevent overeating.

How to reduce stress:

Mindfulness and Meditation: Manage stress effectively by incorporating mindfulness and meditation exercises. These methods help promote relaxation and lower blood pressure.

Hobbies and leisure activities: Encourage activities that people enjoy, such as reading, gardening or listening to music, to relieve stress.

Limit alcohol consumption:

Moderate alcohol consumption is important.

Some studies suggest that moderate alcohol consumption can benefit the cardiovascular system, but excessive alcohol consumption can increase blood pressure.

It encourages moderation or, for some people, complete abstinence.

Quit smoking:

Benefits of Quitting Smoking: Highlights the many health benefits of quitting smoking, including the positive impact on blood pressure. Smoking damages blood vessels and causes high blood pressure.

Enough sleep:

Quality over quantity: Emphasizes the importance of quantity and quality of sleep.
Lack of sleep can have a negative effect on blood pressure.
Establishing a regular sleep routine can help.

Hydration

The importance of drinking water: Staying well hydrated is essential to your overall health.

Although there is limited evidence that hydration is directly related to blood pressure, it is important to maintain an adequate fluid balance.

Regular monitoring:

Home blood pressure monitoring: Encourage people to check their blood pressure at home regularly.

This will help you monitor your progress and provide valuable information to your healthcare professionals.

Taken together, these lifestyle changes create a holistic approach to lowering blood pressure naturally.

It is important to recognize that these changes are interdependent and that a comprehensive strategy is more effective than focusing on one aspect.

Chapter 3
Dietary Choices

Diet plays an important role in lowering blood pressure naturally.
What we eat has a direct impact on our cardiovascular health, and conscious choices can make a significant contribution to blood pressure control.
Let's look at some nutritional strategies you can use for this purpose.

Focus on a balanced diet:

Encourage people to eat a diet that includes a variety of nutritious foods.

A balanced diet provides essential vitamins, minerals and antioxidants for overall health.
The DASH Diet (Diet to Stop High Blood Pressure):

The DASH diet is specifically designed to lower blood pressure.
Examples:

Fruits and vegetables: Rich in potassium, magnesium and fiber.

Whole grains: Rich in fiber and essential nutrients.

Lean proteins: These include fish, poultry, beans and nuts.
Low-fat dairy products: sources of calcium and protein.

Reduce your sodium intake by:

Limit processed foods: Processed and packaged foods are high in sodium. Encourage people to control their salt intake by choosing fresh, unprocessed foods and cooking them at home.

Herbs and spices: Instead of using too much salt, we suggest using herbs and spices to add flavor to your dishes. Increase your intake of potassium-rich foods:

Bananas, oranges, spinach and sweet potatoes: These foods are rich in potassium, which helps balance sodium levels in the body.

Foods rich in magnesium:

Green leafy vegetables, nuts and seeds: Magnesium supports healthy blood vessels and helps regulate blood pressure.
Foods rich in fiber:

Whole grains, fruits, vegetables, and legumes: A high-fiber diet improves heart health by improving cholesterol levels and supporting healthy blood vessels.

Omega-3 fatty acids:

Fatty fish, flax seeds, walnuts: Omega-3 fatty acids have anti-inflammatory effects and help lower blood pressure. Limit saturated and trans fats.

Choose healthy fats: Choose sources of unsaturated fats such as olive oil, avocados and nuts.
Limit saturated and trans fats in processed and fried foods.

Average alcohol consumption:

Moderate amounts of red wine: Some studies suggest that moderate consumption of red wine may benefit the cardiovascular system.

Moderate alcohol consumption is important, but excessive alcohol consumption can raise blood pressure.

Foods rich in calcium:

Low-fat dairy products, leafy greens: Calcium is essential for maintaining strong bones and may play a role in regulating blood pressure.

Track your sugar intake:

Limit added sugar: Excessive sugar consumption has been linked to obesity and other health problems.
It is recommended that you reduce your intake of sugary drinks and processed sweets.

Stay hydrated:

Water as your primary drink: Staying well hydrated is essential to your overall health.
Although water itself has no direct effect on blood pressure, adequate hydration supports overall well-being.

Meal time:

Regular, balanced diet: A regular, balanced diet is recommended to keep blood sugar levels stable. Spreading your food intake throughout the day can help prevent large peaks and valleys in your blood pressure.

Talk to a Registered Dietitian:

Personalized guidance: For people with special nutritional needs or health concerns, a consultation with a registered dietitian can provide personalized guidance on blood pressure management.

This nutritional approach, combined with other lifestyle changes, creates a comprehensive strategy to lower blood pressure naturally.

Chapter 4
Herbal Remedies

Herbal remedies have been studied for their potential to lower blood pressure naturally.

Although these treatments are not a substitute for medical advice or prescription drugs, some herbs have shown promising effects in controlling high blood pressure.

Here are some of them :

Hibiscus:

Benefits: In some studies, hibiscus tea has been shown to lower blood pressure. It is known to act as a natural ACE inhibitor that relaxes blood vessels.

Considerations: Combining hibiscus with certain medications may lower blood pressure excessively, so people taking antihypertensive medications should consult their healthcare provider.

garlic:
Benefits: Garlic has been studied for its ability to lower blood pressure.
It is known to dilate blood vessels and has a mild anticoagulant effect.
Considerations: Garlic supplements may interact with certain medications, including blood thinners.
Be especially careful if you are preparing for surgery.

Olive leaf extract:

Benefits: Antioxidant-rich olive leaf extract has been studied for its cardiovascular benefits, including its ability to lower blood pressure.

Considerations: Although generally considered safe, people with low blood pressure or taking blood pressure medication should monitor their blood pressure closely.

Cinnamon:

Benefits: Cinnamon may have mild antihypertensive effects.

It is also known to have the effect of improving blood sugar control.

Considerations: High doses of cinnamon supplements should be used with caution.

People with liver disease are advised to consult their doctor.

ginger:

Benefits: Ginger has anti-inflammatory properties and helps lower blood pressure by relaxing blood vessels.

Considerations: Ginger may interact with blood thinners and should be used with caution by people with gallstones.

turmeric:

Benefits: Curcumin, the active compound in turmeric, has anti-inflammatory and antioxidant properties that may have positive effects on cardiovascular health.

Considerations: Although generally safe, excessive amounts of turmeric may interfere with the effectiveness of certain medications.

People with gallbladder problems should be cautious.

Flaxseed:
Benefits: Flaxseeds are rich in omega-3 fatty acids, promote cardiovascular health and help regulate blood pressure.
Considerations: When consuming flax seeds, ensure adequate hydration, as their high fiber content can cause digestive problems if not consumed with enough water.

green tea:
Benefits: Green tea contains compounds that have a positive effect on blood pressure.
It is also rich in antioxidants.

Considerations: Although generally safe, drinking too much green tea can cause caffeine-related side effects.
Those who are sensitive to caffeine should be careful.

cat's claws:
Benefits: Cat's claw, an herb derived from a woody vine, has been studied for its effects in lowering blood pressure.
Considerations: Cat's claw may interact with some medications, including antihypertensive medications.
It is recommended to consult a doctor.

It is important to use herbal remedies with caution and be aware of potential drug interactions or existing health conditions.

.

Chapter 5
Exercise And Physical Activity

Exercise and physical activity are an essential part of a natural approach to lowering blood pressure.

Regular physical activity not only benefits overall cardiovascular health, but also plays an important role in controlling and preventing high blood pressure.

Let's take a closer look at why exercise can be a key factor in lowering blood pressure naturally.

Cardiovascular exercises:

Benefits: Participating in aerobic exercise, such as walking, jogging, cycling or swimming, can have a direct effect on blood pressure.
These activities improve cardiovascular health, improve circulation and help the heart work more efficiently.

Recommendation: Get at least 150 minutes of moderate-intensity aerobic exercise per week or 75 minutes of vigorous-intensity exercise seven days a week.

weight training:

Benefits: Resistance or strength training with weights or resistance bands improves overall fitness and helps lower blood pressure.

Recommendation: Include strength training for your major muscle groups at least twice a week.

Flexibility and elasticity:

Benefits: Activities that improve flexibility, such as stretching or yoga, promote relaxation and help reduce stress, which indirectly affects blood pressure.

Recommendation: Add stretching exercises to your daily routine to improve flexibility and overall relaxation.

Consistency and Consistency:

Benefits: Regular exercise is key to long-term blood pressure benefits. Regular physical activity helps keep blood vessels flexible and improves heart function.
Tip: Create a routine that includes a variety of exercises that you're likely to stick to over time.

Strength is important:

Benefit: Any physical activity is better than no physical activity, but high-intensity exercise has the greatest effect on lowering blood pressure.

However, it is very important that individuals choose sustainable activities.

Recommendation: Gradually increase exercise intensity based on fitness level and underlying health conditions.

Adjust your workout intensity:

Benefit: Adjusting exercise intensity allows people to exercise at an appropriate level.
This can be done through methods such as heart rate monitoring or perceived magnitude of exertion.
Recommended: Learn how to measure and monitor exercise intensity to ensure safe and effective exercise.

Integrate physical activity into your daily life:

Benefits: In addition to structured exercise sessions, incorporating physical activity into your daily routine, such as taking the stairs, going for short walks or walking instead of gardening, can improve your overall health.

Recommendation: Find ways to stay active throughout the day, not just during certain exercises.

Personalized approach:

Benefit: Recognize that exercise isn't for everyone. The type, duration and intensity of physical activity may vary according to individual fitness level, preferences and health status.

Recommendation: Consult your healthcare provider or fitness professional to develop an exercise plan tailored to your individual needs and abilities.

Exercises for mind and body:

Benefits: Mental exercises such as Tai Chi and Qigong combine physical activity and relaxation techniques.
These habits help reduce stress and control blood pressure.
Recommendation: Consider mind-body training as part of a holistic approach to physical activity.

Gradual progression:

Benefits: For those starting or returning after a break, gradual progress is important. This reduces the risk of injury and ensures continued participation.

Recommendation: Start with low to moderate intensity exercise and gradually increase the duration and intensity as your condition improves.

Regular, adapted physical activity can be a powerful and natural way to lower blood pressure.
This complements other lifestyle changes and promotes overall cardiovascular health.

Chapter 6
Stress Management Technique

Managing stress is an important part of lowering blood pressure naturally. Chronic stress can contribute to elevated blood pressure, and using effective stress management techniques can have a positive impact on overall cardiovascular health.

Here is a comprehensive review of different stress management strategies:

Mindfulness Meditation:

Benefits: Mindfulness meditation involves being present in the present moment and being fully present in that moment.

Regular exercise has been associated with lower stress levels and lower blood pressure.

Practical tip: Try practicing mindfulness meditation for a few minutes every day.

Develop calmness by focusing on your breath, your emotions, or a specific mantra.

Deep breathing exercises:

Benefits: Deep breathing activates the body's relaxation response, reduces stress hormones and creates feelings of calm.

It helps lower blood pressure.

Practical tip: Practice diaphragmatic breathing by inhaling deeply through your nose, expanding your abdomen and exhaling slowly through your mouth.

Progressive muscle relaxation (PMR):

Benefits: PMR involves systematically tensing and then relaxing different muscle groups to promote general relaxation and reduce tension.
Practical tip: Find a quiet place and tense your muscles, starting with your toes, then relax.
Work each muscle group in turn to get to the top.

yoga:

Benefits: Yoga combines physical postures, controlled breathing and meditation to promote relaxation and reduce stress.

Regular exercise has been associated with improved cardiovascular health.

Practical tip: Join a local class or take an online yoga session.

For soothing benefits, choose a gentle or restorative style of yoga.

Biological feedback:

Advantages: Biofeedback uses electronic monitoring to inform and monitor physiological processes.

It helps manage stress-related symptoms, including blood pressure.

Practical tip: Work with a qualified biofeedback therapist to learn how to manage physiological responses such as heart rate and muscle tension.

Featured Image:

Benefits: Guided imagery uses mental imagery to induce feelings of calm and relaxation.This helps reduce stress and in turn lowers blood pressure.
Practical tip: Listen to a guided video or create your own mental image of a peaceful and calm scene when you feel stressed.

Tai Chi:

Benefits: Tai Chi is a gentle martial art that combines slow, flowing movements with deep breathing and meditation. It has been associated with

reduced stress and improved cardiovascular health.
Practical tip: Consider taking a Tai Chi class or watching an instructional video to incorporate this exercise into your daily routine.

Regular sport:

Benefit: Physical activity reduces severe stress. It releases endorphins, improves mood and helps the body cope more effectively with stress.
Practical advice: Find an activity you enjoy - walking, running, swimming, dancing - and include it in your daily routine.

journalism:

Benefit: Writing down your thoughts and feelings provides freedom and insight. Journaling can be a useful tool for coping with stress and managing your emotions.

Practical advice: Take time every day to write down your experiences, thoughts and feelings.

This can be done through traditional magazines or digital platforms.

Social support:

Benefit: Sharing your concerns with friends, family, or a support network can help you gain emotional stability and manage stress.

Practical advice: Build strong social connections.

Spend regular time with loved ones and talk openly about your feelings.

Time management:

Benefit: Effective time management reduces overwhelm and stress.
Prioritizing tasks and setting realistic goals can help you live a balanced lifestyle.
Practical tip: Use tools like a calendar or to-do list to organize your time.
Learn to say no when necessary and delegate tasks when possible.

Nature and outdoor activities:

Benefit: Spending time in nature has been linked to reduced levels of stress. Whether it's a walk in the park or a hike in the mountains, connecting with nature can have a calming effect.

Practical tip: Include outdoor activities in your daily routine.
Even a short walk in a nearby natural environment can bring about positive changes.

Laughter Therapy:

Benefit: Laughter triggers the release of endorphins, which create feelings of happiness. It also helps reduce stress hormones and lower blood pressure.

Practical advice: Engage in activities that bring you joy and laughter, such as watching funny movies, going to comedy shows, or spending time with funny friends.

Music therapy:

Benefits: Listening to music has a calming effect on the nervous system, reduces stress and promotes relaxation.

Practical tip: Create a playlist of soothing music and incorporate it into your daily routine.
Explore genres known to have calming effects, such as classical or instrumental music.

Cognitive behavioral therapy (CBT):

Benefits: CBT is a therapeutic approach that helps people identify and change negative thought patterns and behaviors that contribute to stress.

Practical tip: Work with an experienced therapist to learn CBT techniques to improve stress management and coping strategies.

It's important to remember that coping with stress is a personal journey and what works for one person may not work for another.
It's often helpful to experiment with different methods and find a combination that suits your tastes and lifestyle. Consistent use of stress management techniques is important to achieve long-term benefits in lowering blood pressure naturally.

Chapter 7
Sleep And Resting

Sleep plays an important role in maintaining overall health and has a significant impact on blood pressure. Chronic sleep deprivation or lack of sleep can lead to high blood pressure and other cardiovascular problems.

Below is a comprehensive overview of the relationship between sleep and blood pressure and strategies for lowering blood pressure naturally by improving sleep.

Sleep time and blood pressure:

Research findings: Studies have shown that both long and short sleep are associated with increased blood pressure. The optimal amount of sleep for cardiovascular health is generally about 7 to 9 hours per night for most adults.

Sleep quality is important:

Impact on blood pressure: In addition to the amount of sleep you get, the quality of your sleep is also very important. Conditions such as sleep apnea, insomnia, or restless legs syndrome can disrupt sleep patterns and cause high blood pressure.

Treating sleep disorders: Identifying and treating sleep disorders by consulting with your healthcare provider can be an important step in managing your blood pressure naturally.

Sleep and circadian rhythm:

Natural biological clock: The body's internal clock, or circadian rhythm, regulates the sleep-wake cycle and affects blood pressure.

Blood pressure usually follows a diurnal pattern of falling at night and rising in the morning.

Blood disorders and high blood pressure: Circadian rhythm disorders, such as irregular sleep patterns or shift work, can cause high blood pressure. Maintaining a regular sleep schedule helps maintain a healthy circadian rhythm.

How sleep deprivation affects stress hormones:

Cortisol levels: Lack of sleep can increase levels of stress hormones, especially cortisol.High levels of cortisol are associated with increased blood pressure.

Reduce stress through sleep: Prioritizing adequate, quality sleep helps regulate stress hormones and promotes a healthy response to daily stressors.

Hormonal balance related to sleep:

Growth hormone release: Good sleep is essential for the release of growth hormone, which plays a role in maintaining the integrity of the cardiovascular system.

Adequate sleep helps with hormonal balance and overall health.

Sleep hygiene rules:

Create a comfortable sleep environment: Creating a comfortable sleep environment includes factors such as keeping the room cool and dark, reducing noise and investing in a comfortable mattress and pillows.

Consistent bedtime routine: Creating a consistent bedtime routine tells your body it's time to rest, promoting relaxation and better sleep.

Limit stimulants before bed.

Caffeine and blood pressure: Caffeine can temporarily increase blood pressure.
Limiting caffeine consumption, especially in the hours before bed, can help improve sleep quality.

Avoid overeating and alcohol: Overeating and drinking close to bedtime can also interfere with sleep.Choosing a light dinner and moderate alcohol consumption can help improve your sleep.

Regular physical activity and sleep:

Exercise and sleep quality: Regular physical activity is associated with improved sleep quality.
Participating in aerobic exercise, such as walking or running, can have a positive effect on both blood pressure and sleep.

Timing of exercise: Regular exercise is beneficial, but vigorous activity close to bedtime can have a stimulating effect and affect sleep.
Try to finish any vigorous exercise a few hours before bed.

Mindfulness and relaxation techniques:

Reduce stress for better sleep: Mindfulness exercises, meditation, and relaxation exercises can help reduce stress and develop a calm mind that can help you sleep better.

Incorporate relaxation into your sleep routine: Incorporating relaxation techniques into your sleep routine can signal your body that it's time to rest.

Create a positive mindset about sleep:

Associate bedtime with rest: To develop a positive mindset about sleep, you need to associate bedtime with rest and rejuvenation rather than stress or anxiety.

Addressing sleep anxiety: Cognitive-behavioral therapy for insomnia (CBT-I) can be an effective approach for people with sleep-related anxiety.

Sleep and blood pressure:

Short naps: Short naps during the day are associated with potential blood pressure benefits. However, prolonged or irregular sleep patterns can interfere with a good night's sleep.

Regular sleep patterns: If you sleep, aim for short, regular periods of sleep during the day to avoid disrupting your nighttime sleep.

Professional guidance:

Anyone with ongoing sleep problems or blood pressure concerns should talk to their healthcare provider.

A sleep study or evaluation may be recommended to identify and address underlying problems.

Improving the quality and duration of sleep is a key, natural strategy for managing blood pressure.

It's about adopting consistent sleep habits, eliminating sleep disturbances, and creating an environment conducive to restful sleep.

As with any health-related change, it's important to consult a healthcare professional for individualized advice and to rule out any conditions that may be affecting your sleep or blood pressure.

Chapter 8
Monitoring And Maintaining Blood Pressure

Controlling and maintaining blood pressure plays an important role in natural approaches to treating high blood pressure. Regular monitoring provides insight into the effectiveness of lifestyle changes and allows for timely corrections.

Below is a comprehensive review of monitoring and maintenance strategies to lower blood pressure naturally.

Check your blood pressure at home:
Advantages: Regular home monitoring gives you a complete picture of your blood pressure trends.

This allows people to take an active role in their own health.

Choosing a blood pressure monitor: Choose a reliable blood pressure monitor for your home and follow proper measurement techniques. Correspondence between time zone and observing conditions increases accuracy.

To keep a blood pressure record:

Benefits: Keeping a blood pressure record helps you track patterns and identify factors that affect your blood pressure.
This provides valuable information for discussion with your doctor.

Record lifestyle factors: Record details of your diet, exercise, stress levels and sleep patterns in a diary to see if these correlate with your blood pressure levels.

Regular health checks:
Significance: Enables comprehensive assessment of cardiovascular health.
These visits may include taking your blood pressure, blood tests, and discussing your lifestyle habits.
Collaborative approach: We work with your healthcare professional to set individual blood pressure goals and discuss strategies to reach and maintain your goals naturally.

Medication Management:

Tips for Health Care Providers: For people prescribed high blood pressure medication, it is very important to follow the prescribed regimen.

Regular check-ups with your doctor will ensure that your medications are effective and well tolerated.

Open Communication: Discuss any concerns or side effects with your healthcare provider.

Depending on the individual's response, medication adjustments or lifestyle recommendations may be necessary.

Dietary changes:

Long-term commitment: Adopting a heart-healthy diet is not a short-term solution.
Continuous efforts are needed to change the diet, such as the DASH diet, which is rich in fruits, vegetables and whole grains.

Regular evaluation: Regularly evaluate and adjust food choices based on personal preferences and health goals.
Consider speaking with a registered dietitian for personalized guidance.

Regular sport:

Consistency is the key.
Regular physical activity is a lifelong commitment.

Consistency in your exercise routine provides lasting cardiovascular benefits and supports blood pressure control.

Regular reviews: We regularly re-evaluate our training to ensure it remains challenging and enjoyable. Adjustments may be required to accommodate changes in fitness level or preferences.

Practice stress management:

Integrate into your daily life: Stress management techniques such as mindfulness and deep breathing should be incorporated into your daily life. Regular exercise naturally increases the blood pressure lowering effect.

Explore new techniques: We are constantly exploring new ways to manage stress to keep the experience fresh and exciting. Consider activities such as yoga, tai chi or progressive muscle relaxation.

Sleep hygiene:

Prioritize quality sleep. Maintaining good sleep hygiene is an ongoing effort.
A consistent sleep pattern, a suitable sleep environment and the elimination of sleep disturbances contribute to improved overall health.

Periodic sleep assessment: regularly assess the quality and duration of your sleep. If you're having trouble sleeping, see your healthcare provider to identify and address the root cause.

Weight maintenance:

Balanced approach: Achieving and maintaining a healthy weight requires a balanced approach to diet and exercise.
Crash diets or extreme exercise regimes are neither sustainable nor beneficial in the long term.

Regular review: Review your weight management strategy regularly.
Changes in lifestyle, metabolism or health may require adjustments.

Support and social responsibility:

Get Your Loved Ones Involved: Get your friends and family involved in lowering your blood pressure naturally.
Social support and accountability can be motivating factors in maintaining healthy habits.

Regular Check-ins: Schedule regular check-ins with your health buddy or support group to discuss progress, challenges, and successes.
Celebrate success together.

Attention and reflection:

Regular reflection: Take time to regularly reflect on your lifestyle choices and how they affect your blood pressure.
Conscious awareness leads to informed decision making.

Adjust your goals: Review your health goals regularly and adjust them as your priorities, preferences or health status change.
Additional knowledge:

Stay informed: Stay up to date with new research and information about high blood pressure management.
Secondary education enables people to make informed decisions about their health.

See your healthcare provider: If you notice new findings or concerns during your routine checkup, discuss them with your healthcare provider.Work together to incorporate solid strategies into your overall plan.

Celebrating Achievements:
Recognize achievements: Celebrate milestones and achievements in blood pressure management.
Positive reinforcement reinforces the value of sustainable lifestyle changes.
Set new goals: Once your blood pressure improves, it may be a good idea to set new health goals to stay motivated and accomplished.

Adapting to life changes:

Flexibility: Life circumstances can change and require lifestyle changes. Be flexible and adjust your strategy to accommodate changes in your work schedule, family responsibilities, or other factors.

Get help: If you're making a big change in your life, get advice from your healthcare provider or support network to help you manage potential problems while staying focused on managing your blood pressure.

Developing a holistic approach:

Integrated health perspective: Considers blood pressure management as part of a holistic approach to health.

Consider the interconnectedness of physical, mental and emotional well-being.

Balance and Harmony: Strive for balance that promotes harmony in various aspects of life.

Overall health promotes stable blood pressure control.

In conclusion, it is clear that controlling and maintaining blood pressure requires a total and lifelong commitment to health.

Regular evaluations, working with your healthcare provider, and ongoing lifestyle changes provide a comprehensive and effective approach to managing high blood pressure.

Combining natural strategies such as dietary changes, regular exercise, stress management, and quality sleep can contribute to overall cardiovascular health and wellness.

Conclusion

As we conclude your journey through "How To Lower Your Blood Pressure Naturally, we sincerely congratulate you on taking positive steps to live a healthy and harmonious life.

In these pages, we've explored the complex dance of lifestyle choices, mindful practices, and natural strategies that contribute to optimal blood pressure levels.

Let us say goodbye and consider the meaning of our expedition. This guide is based on the belief that true healing comes from a holistic approach that recognizes the interconnectedness of body, mind, and spirit.

The promise of managing your blood pressure naturally is more than just a regimen.

It's about embracing a lifestyle that aligns with your body's innate wisdom.

Remember,The journey doesn't end here.
Follow through with every conscious choice you make.
Whether you're enjoying nutritious food, engaging in heart-warming exercise, practicing mindful relaxation, or fostering meaningful connections, these are the notes that make up the symphony of well-being.

As you move forward, see this conclusion not as an end point, but as an invitation to continue the harmonious rhythm you have cultivated.

The power to lower your blood pressure is naturally within you and exists through the choices you make every day.
Embrace the journey, appreciate your health and enjoy a happy life.